The 5 Day Watermelon Only Cleanse - How to Use Watermelons to Help Cleanse And Heal Your Body Naturally

How to cleanse and remove stagnant mucu

Some reported benefits of this cleanse:

Lose weight — many have seen 7-10 lbs o

Move and clean the lymphatic system (improve your immune health).

Improve kidney filtration and build self-esteem.

Will you have the courage to take the 5-day watermelon challenge ?

Welcome to the best-tasting detox on earth.

This is a pathway to a new you. It's just 5 days and it's enough time to give you a taste of a healthier you. It is a way to build self-love and self-discipline. To build self-esteem and self-respect, because 5 days is not too long a period but it's enough to show you the potential of what choices you have with foods to make yourself better physically and mentally.

It's going to help you lose weight as well, but more importantly, it's going to show you how to cleanse your body so that it works better and heals and repairs itself faster.

This is an action book, not a theoretical one, and you will become the actual proof of the cleansing and healing properties of a watermelon-only cleanse

So let's begin.

Before We Start: Here Is A Medical Disclaimer.

This book is not about diseases but about natural healing. Diseases to me are concepts or names of symptoms of a deep underlying cause and in natural healing we don't address the effects only the root cause. So we don't treat, cure, diagnose in natural healing. So this book is not about treating, diagnosing or curing but about the body to a place where it can better take care of itself, it's about getting well and healthy. That being said, always see your doctor to diagnose, treat or cure a disease.

So all content found in this book including: text, images, audio, or other formats were created for informational purposes only. The content is not intended to be a substitute for professional medical advice, diagnosis, or treatment. Always seek the advice of your physician or other qualified health provider with any questions you may have regarding a medical condition. Never disregard professional medical advice or delay in seeking it because of something you have read on it in this book.

If you think you may have a medical emergency, call your doctor, go to the emergency department, or call 911 immediately. The author does not recommend or endorse any specific tests, physicians, products, procedures, opinions, or other information that may be mentioned on here. Reliance on any information provided here is solely at your own risk.

The Content in this book is provided on an "as is" basis. Use at your own risk

Why I wrote this book

I wrote this book because I know there are lots of people trying to improve their health but don't fully understand how to do so. So I wrote this book so you understand how the body actually works and how to get the glands, organs and cells healthy.

I am only showing you what I know works. And if you try using the knowledge I share, you will see the body's true potential as a self-healer.

We all love watermelon. It's sweet, it smells delicious and it's refreshing, but did you know it has healing properties? It has been used in Chinese medicine for thousands of years, and I am going to show you how to use it effectively.

There are some major benefits of watermelons, according to Chinese medicine:

(1) Heart health — watermelon is known to be helpful in preventing strokes and heart attacks.

(2) It is deemed helpful in decreasing and normalizing blood pressure.

(3) It boosts sex drive.

(4) It plays an important role in preventing cancer, due to its lycopene content (lycopene is acknowledged in its ability to prevent cancer).

(5) It improves eyesight due to its high vitamin C and A content.

(6) Watermelon is hydrating, as it contains alkaline water. Ninety-two percent of its volume is alkaline water; it is used traditionally for the relief of stomach ailments such as ulcers.

(7) It reduces halitosis (bad breath).

(8) It's a great way to clean and strengthen the kidneys. It helps to clean the urinary tract, kidneys and bladder. It helps resolve UTIs and kidney stones.

(9) It's helpful in fighting gout.

(10) Watermelon juice is a great natural energy drink.

Why watermelon? Watermelon is a berry; its scientific name is Citrullus lanatus and it's an amazing healing fruit. It's astringent (good at moving the lymph system), it's hydrating (it contains water, which makes it easier to hydrate cells) and it's alkalizing to the cells.

Here is the average nutrition found in a melon.

A 1-cup (100 grams) serving of watermelon provides:

Calories: 30
Carbs: 8 grams
Fiber: 1.4 grams
Protein: 1 gram
Fat: 0.2 grams
Vitamin C: 13% of the recommended daily intake (RDI)
Vitamin A: 11% of the RDI
Potassium: 3% of the RDI
Iron: 1% of the RDI
Magnesium: 2% of the RDI
% based on a 2000-calorie diet

Watermelon is one of the least obstructive foods to the human body.

Why?

Watermelons are easy to digest. They take 15-20 minutes to digest.

Watermelon contains lots of water and a small amount of fiber — both of which are important for healthy and quick digestion. Fiber can provide bulk for your stool, while the water it contains helps keep your digestive tract moving efficiently.

Why we get unhealthy

The cause of man's ills is acidosis. This means as a species we are eating the wrong foods. When we eat foods alien to the human body, the body will tend to produce excess mucus, and this excess mucus, if it does not move, will become stagnant and tends to hold metabolic waste. This waste is acidic, and acids accumulate, and if not removed, they create a state of acidosis. Acids are corrosive, they burn, they dehydrate and they will affect the function of cells, tissues, organs and glands. They create ill health.

Why do certain foods create acidosis?

The human species is a frugivore (fruit eater). The proof is that we are closest in species to apes and they are frugivores in their natural environment. We are not carnivores and we are not herbivores either. We certainly don't look like a cat or a horse. So it makes sense that we eat the foods designed for the human body.

More proof lies with the observation that if you put any human from any part of the world on a fruit diet, they will become healthier.

Fruits are the least obstructive foods you can eat. They are mucusless and alkaline as well.

Plus, fruits are the only foods on the planet that are able to move your lymphatic system and help open up all the elimination channels of the body (the kidneys, the digestive system, the skin and the lungs).

The lymphatic system is your main immune system. It is the system that keeps you healthy. And when you consume foods like cooked foods, protein and starches, these foods will acidify and stagnate the lymphatic system. These foods are complex chemistry foods and when they are broken down, the waste that remains in the process is acidic. These wastes have to be removed by the lymphatic system, but they slow down and stagnate the lymphatic system. Acids will also stimulate mucus production in an attempt to buffer these acids, and this excess mucus can affect the function of cells, tissues and organs.

Think of your lymphatic system as a sewer system, and this sewer system is in every cell. Its job among other things is to remove waste from your cells, and if this system gets clogged, your cells are not going to be able to function properly and you will tend to develop health issues.

Fruits also offer astringency, which is a pulling or drying out action that's needed to keep the lymph system moving and healthy. A healthy immune system means good health.

Detoxification

We use detoxification to cleanse the body.

Detoxification is a natural process that the body uses to cleanse itself, but the problem is when we eat foods that obstruct the function of the body; the body can't undergo the process of detoxification (its natural cleansing process) easily or at all. Detoxification is cellular purification.

Detoxification is not a diet; it's a natural cleansing process. If we consumed a fruitarian diet, the process of detoxification would be easier, but we eat abnormally (we eat the wrong foods, we eat too often, and cook our foods). This is affecting natural detoxification and therefore wrecking our health.

Achieving detoxification means eating the right foods and putting your body in an environment that allows it to self-heal or clean itself. It also means leaving behind the bad foods we have been conditioned to consume, along with the frequency at which we've been conditioned to eat.

We use detoxification to help the body get better.

No one expects you to become a fruitarian, but to cleanse the body, a fruit cleanse is needed. And you can always go back and add balance to your diet when you're done healing yourself with this regenerative detoxification cleanse.

Understanding simple chemistry

There are two sides to chemistry.

Acid and base. Acids are damaging, drying, abrasive and dehydrating, and they damage tissue and cause ill health. On the opposite side, a balanced alkaline (base) chemistry nurtures, hydrates and heals. The body is predominantly on the alkaline (base) side, but when we eat foods that are acidic, we put the body a bit more to the acidic side. This acidity is what we call acidosis.

Acidosis stimulates excess mucus production in the body. If this excess mucus production is stagnant, it will damage or affect the function of tissue, organ and glands and cause health issues.

Part of the reason why you are not healthy is because there is a compromise in the function of glands, organs and systems of your body.

And what causes this compromise is acidosis, and acidosis is caused by eating the wrong foods. These foods tend to acidify the body, which in turn affects the lymph system and kidneys. These glands are affected by stagnant mucus and acids that alter the function of the cells, tissues, organs and glands, which can affect the function and health of the whole body.

When the body is free of mucus and acids, there is abundant and free flow of energy (which is defined as blood flow, lymph flow and nerve flow).

When there is healthy energy flow in the body, there is ease in its function and health. However, when these energy flows are obstructed with mucus and acids, there will be disruption in the function of the body (disease).

The Energy Flows of the Body

In detoxification there are 3 major energy flows we broadly recognize: nerve flow, lymph flow and blood flow. Nerve flow is needed to allow communication between cells of the body. Lymph flow is part of the immune system of the body; it's what removes waste from your cells. Blood flow is what feeds the cells and gives oxygen to cells. If any of these energy flows are blocked or interrupted, the body is not going to function properly.

For instance, a blockage in lymph flow can apply pressure to nerve flow or blood flow.

A blockage in nerve flow can affect blood flow, resulting in poor nutrition to the cells, and can negatively affect nerve flow, resulting in weak communication between cells.

A blockage in blood flow can affect nerve flow and lymph flow, as tissue and cells won't survive without the other two.

The fact is, proper energy flow equals good health.

The fruit diet is a tool we use together with herbs to open or clean these energy pathways.

And the watermelon-only diet is one of my favorites for improving energy flow.

Bad health is all "cause and effect."

Your health issues are caused by your eating the wrong foods, which causes obstructions, which causes a blockage of energy flow, which causes health issues.

More specifically, you are what you eat. If you eat foods that are obstructive to the human body (cause), you will experience disease (effect). It's that simple.

So most health issues are symptoms of an obstruction in the body. Unless you got a virus or some other pathogen, you did not "catch a disease" — you manifested it with your diet and lifestyle choices.

Even eating a conventional "healthy diet" is obstructive to health, as it contains mucus-forming and acidic foods (protein, starches, processed foods and even cooked foods).

The good news is that if you recognize this cause-and-effect principle, you can turn things around with the right tools: fruits and herbs.

Its called taking responsibility.

Raw Maraby's 3 universal steps to getting the body healthy.

Step #1: Change the diet and eat the least obstructive or nonobstructive food, i.e., fruit. In this book, we are going to be using watermelon.

Step #2: Use herbs to clean and strengthen the structure and function of cells.

Step #3: Give the detoxification process time. It took you years to manifest this ill health, but the good news is that it will take you a fraction of that time to turn things around.

Understanding the major organs, glands and systems for an effective cleanse.

Let me explain the major systems and organs of the human body in a very simple way.

The lymphatic system

The lymph system is your immune system or your "sewer" system and its job is to remove acidic waste from your cells to the lymph nodes and then to the kidneys and if it does not work well, the Lymph system backs up and these acids affect the function of the cells (tissue, organ and glands) the bowels and the kidneys-

Adrenals

Why we need healthy Adrenals

Why you need your adrenals in good shape

1. They control the kidneys (the doorway to health)

2. They control the autonomic nervous system and movements like breathing and peristalsis. They produce neurotransmitters to control body functions - Neurotransmitters are messengers that transmit a message from nerve cells to other cells (nerve cells, muscle cells and or gland cells)

3. They fight inflammation. Your adrenal glands produce hormones that help regulate your metabolism, immune system, blood pressure, response to stress and other essential functions.

Adrenal glands work to produce cortisol, which helps control the body's use of fats, proteins and carbohydrates; suppresses inflammation; regulates blood pressure; increases blood sugar; and can also decrease bone formation.

This hormone also controls the sleep/wake cycle. It is released during times of stress to help your body get an energy boost and better handle an emergency situation.

Adrenals produce Aldosterone, which plays a central role in regulating blood pressure and certain electrolytes (sodium and potassium). Aldosterone controls the kidneys by using signals to the kidneys, which gets the kidneys to absorb more sodium into the bloodstream and at the same time release expelled potassium into urine. This means that adrenals produce aldosterone, which helps regulate the blood pH by controlling the sodium and potassium balance in the blood - it's an alkalizer for the blood.

Adrenals produce DHEA and Androgenic Steroids

These hormones are male hormones. They are precursor hormones that can be converted in the ovaries into estrogen and in the testes into androgens.

They are the fight or flight glands.

They produce Epinephrine (Adrenaline) and Norepinephrine (Noradrenaline)

The adrenals control the hormones that induce "the flight or fight response". The major hormones secreted by the adrenal glands to initiate the flight or fight response are epinephrine (adrenaline) and norepinephrine (noradrenaline), these hormones
Can increase the heart rate this will in turn increase blood flow to the muscles and to the brain. It also helps assist with sugar metabolism. These hormones also help control the contracting of the blood vessels and help maintain the right blood pressure and increase it in response to a stress situation

Symptoms of poor adrenals might include anxiety, panic attacks, moody, poor breathing, poor bowel movements and low energy.

The kidneys

Your kidneys are located in the region of your lower back. You have two of them. One on the left and one on the right.

What do kidneys do?

I like to think of the kidneys as the washing machine for your blood but more importantly for your lymphatic system. The kidneys are the sewer plant of the body. The kidneys filter out metabolic waste from the lymphatic system. The kidneys dump the waste to the bladder and are excreted as urine.

The kidneys also help: control water levels, regulate blood pressure, red blood cell production, as well as the levels of calcium and other minerals in the body.

Kidneys are a crucial part of the health of your body for the simple reason that if you don't remove the lymphatic waste, this acidic waste will stimulate excess mucus and stagnate and begin to damage and affect the function of your glands, organs and tissues.

The endocrine glands

The endocrine glands tell your cells what to do and how to function via hormone production.

There are a few endocrine glands in the body, these are the: Adrenal gland, Thyroid gland, Pituitary gland, Parathyroid gland, Pancreas, Pineal gland, Hypothalamus. Ovary and Thymus

The pituitary gland is the master gland of the endocrine system. Its job is to make and release hormones that direct and control other endocrine glands

The Digestive system — Bowels and GI tract.

The digestive system is made up of all the parts of the body that work together to help turn the food and liquids consumed into the nutrients, energy and building blocks needed to repair, fuel and build the body. This is housed In the GI tract.

Your GI tract compromises everything from
The tip of your tongue to your anus and connects every single organ in some way. It's the core of the body and essential to health.

When you put something in your mouth or even smell it, taste it or touch it, it starts the digestive process. Saliva is produced in the mouth to start the digestive process.

Saliva makes the food soft then it's pushed to your esophagus moves the food to the stomach
The stomach is like a processor of the food eaten, it breaks down the food into nutrients that can be absorbed and broken down by the small intestines.

The small intestines are aided by the pancreas, liver, and gallbladder. The pancreas helps digest fats and protein, the liver and gallbladder uses bile to help absorb it into the bloodstream.

The nutrients once absorbed by the small intestines can be sent to the bloodstream to feed the cells. These nutrients also make it to the liver to be transformed or transmuted into what the body needs.

All leftover food that is not made use of ends up in the large intestines.

The nutrient-rich blood makes its way to the liver for further processing. The liver's job is to filter out any harmful substance or waste - it turns the waste into bile. The liver determines how many nutrients and what nutrients go to the parts of the body, and also how many nutrients will be stored for later use.

The large intestines is where all left over processed waste from the food you ate is sent to, to be eliminated via the rectum and anus. The appendix is attached to the large intestines and is the main lymph node of the colon. (It's not a useless part of the colon).

The waste that hits the large intestines and passes through to the colon where the body has a last chance of absorbing water and nutrients - the absorption of water leaves the waste a solid where it is pushed to the rectum to come out as stool. Stools come out through the anus.

For optimal health the digestive system
Has to be healthy and it's kept healthy by using the right foods and herbs to address the pancreas, liver, intestines and colon.

When you use fruits it takes 15-30 minutes to digest -the fruits are not obstructive and act like scrubbers and clean as well as nurture and provide nutrition. You have food that is not only cleaning but also healing.

The colon must be kept light and free flowing and not constipated. Eating cooked starches, processed foods and proteins take a long time to digest and this creates obstructions to the digestive system, which leads to health issues. Consuming fruits (watermelon in this case) offers the body a break as well as an opportunity to cleanse itself.

I call these parts fabulous five and later on I will show you how to use herbs to help you strengthen these parts of your body.

<u>Mucus</u>

Mucus is a part of the lymphatic system -the lymphatic system is a system that is in every single cell in our bodies all hundred trillion cells of our body will eat by the blood and is therefore nourished by the blood and it will eliminate waste by the lymphatic system.

The lymphatic system is the main immune system in the body but in this scenario here it's also the main sewer system in the body so its job is to transfer acids to the lymph nodes where it's converted to lesser acids and then to the kidneys where it's eliminated out of the body.

If the kidneys are not working properly and are not filtering out metabolic waste the sewer system (lymph) will back up and in this backing up it will hold metabolic waste and acids and these acids will burn tissue, organs and glands and will affect the function of cells organs and tissue.

So what happens is that when you're eating processed foods, starches, and animal products for a period of time (it could take years and decades to backup) it creates a dysfunction of organs, glands and tissue.

So if you want to get healthy, the proper way to do it is to cleanse the body of stagnant mucus and acids. This is done with fruits and herbs.

So in summary, this is a 5-day watermelon-only cleanse. In my opinion it's one of the most powerful and effective cleanses you can use. You are going to feel great and feel and see the power of fruits. Let's begin.

How To Check For Kidney Filtration

How often do you check your urine to see if your kidneys are filtering properly or not? If you're like most people, the answer is: not often enough.

Here's an easy way to determine whether or not your kidneys are filtering properly or not. When your kidneys are filtering well you will see sediments in your urine; cloud like particles or mucus strands. The best time to do this is when you use the bathroom first thing in the morning.

Filtration is one of the keys to health because it shows that your body is getting rid of metabolic waste from your hundred trillion cells.

When they aren't being removed from your body they will become problems for you in the future because it will accumulate and you will become backed up. These acids will start to burn through your tissues, organs and glands, which could lead to countless ailments and conditions.

If you find that you're not filtering properly you want to do a fruit cleanse with some dry fasting. The fruits will get your lymph moving and the dry fasting will help with your kidneys.

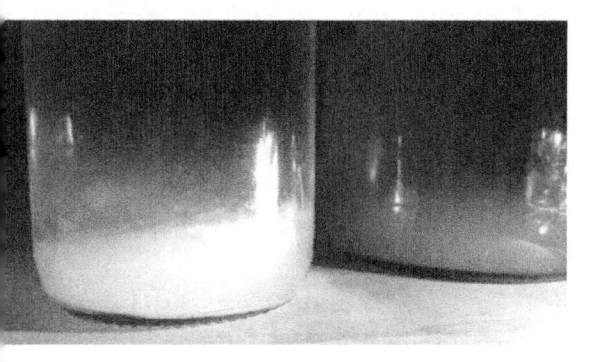

This is what filtration looks like (see picture above) for most it won't be as much but you need to see some sediment in it.

Below I have listed the ingredients for the herbal formulas I indicated above. You can make your own or simply get it on my website. If you can't get all the herbs for each formula you can use what you can get your hands on.

Use bowel strength tincture if you are constipated - use it 5-7 times a day until you get movement

TRANSITION BEFORE YOU BEGIN

If you're coming from a standard American diet, you need a few days to transition to the watermelon-only cleanse.

We transition to make it easier for the body to adapt and function better on the cleanse. The transition also lessens the healing crisis that one may experience on a cleanse.

Here is how to transition:

You're going to have fruit for breakfast; you can have any kind of fruit you prefer.

For lunch you have fruits as well, and for dinner you can have some steamed vegetables or a big raw salad.

If that is too aggressive for you, you can make it less aggressive as follows:
Breakfast: fruits (you can have any)
Lunch: a big raw salad
Dinner: steamed vegetables.

You are going to want to eat like this for a week, or at the very least, two or three days before you jump into the watermelon-only cleanse.

The watermelon-only cleanse

In this cleanse all you are doing is simply replacing all your meals with fresh watermelon and watermelon juice. Now when I say replace all your meals, I mean replace all food and all meals! This means forgoing snacks like coffee, nuts, and anything else you put into your mouth.

While drinking coffee or caffeinated teas does not make a meal, it's still an ingestion of matter and it affects the chemistry of the body. So just to make it very clear, on this cleanse you eat nothing but watermelon. This limitation does not include water, herbal tinctures and teas.

Anything else that you normally consume is going to be replaced by watermelon.

That is how simple it is, and for each meal, you're going to have two or three cups of watermelon per meal, and you can have three to five meals in a day.

THE PLAN

The two tools you need for this cleanse:

1. Watermelon
2. Herbs.

You are simply replacing all your meals with watermelon or watermelon juice. You'll also be using herbs, called the fabulous 5, which I will list below in the herb section of this book.

How much watermelon do you need?

You won't need more than one large watermelon per day (18-20 pounds or 9 kgs).

You will need five large watermelons or eight small watermelons for the five-day cleanse.

The cleanse is very simple. Let me summarize:

All you are doing is simply replacing all the meals you currently eat (including snacks) with fresh watermelon and watermelon juice.

By this I mean that you eat nothing but watermelon for breakfast, lunch and dinner - the key is to eat small frequent meals every two to three hours.

For the next five days, you don't eat any food but watermelon.

Here us what it looks like:

Breakfast after 11am: watermelon (2-3 cups)
Lunch: watermelon (2-3 cups)
Dinner: watermelon (2-3 cups)

The above is just an example — you can eat a small watermelon meal when you are hungry.

You can eat and juice your watermelon as a meal if you wish.

If you are hungry in between breakfast, lunch and dinner, eat more watermelon.

However do not eat too late or you will tend to need to urinate, and this will likely disrupt your sleep. Eat your last watermelon two hours before bed.

You want small, frequent meals. Consume watermelon every two hours. If you are not hungry, don't force yourself to eat.

The best time to consume watermelon is alone *or 30-45 minutes before or after a meal. If you mix with food, it digests quickly and ferments on undigested food, causing gas.*

As this is a watermelon-only cleanse, the above tip is a good point to know about watermelon if you were eating it as part of a regular diet.

Q: How much watermelon should I consume?

A: The amount of watermelon to be eaten per serving is 2-4 cups. If juice, 1-2 cups per serving. The key is to not overeat or under eat. Eat until satisfied and keep the belly half full.

How to speed up the process of detoxification on the watermelon-only cleanse:

Add some intermittent dry fasting to it.

In this modification, you perform a 14-to-18-hour dry fast (no food and no water) and then you break the fast with 16 to 20 ounces of watermelon juice. After the juice, wait 30 minutes, then eat your watermelon meal and repeat the process, or next day go on a watermelon-only diet.

You can experiment with it to see what sequence you enjoy between the hours of fasting and the watermelon-only diet.

Forms of watermelon available (seeds, juice, rind and flesh)

Using the seeds of the watermelon

The seeds are well known to work as a diuretic and may even help soothe and relieve urinary tract infections.[1]

The seeds are to be ground or crushed and used with boiling water, as you would make a tea, in a ratio of 1 teaspoon of ground seeds to a pint of boiling water.[2]

How to use the seeds

Place 1-2 teaspoons of dried crushed watermelon seeds in a coffee mug and fill it with 16-42 ounces of boiling water. Let it steep, and when cool enough, strain and drink it.

You can also put 2-3 tablespoons of the crushed seeds into a large glass jar and add boiling water to it. Let it cool down and sip it all day. (This is called micro-dosing.)

The seed powder can also be eaten. You can also use seeds in tincture form as well.

You can also use fresh seeds

How to prepare watermelon seeds:

Pick the seeds from the freshly cut watermelon and air or sun dry them for a day or two. You can also dehydrate them (temperature setting should be below 115° F). Once dry, grind the seeds in a coffee grinder or any way you choose.

Once ground, store in a dry place like a glass jar (it has to be 100% dry or it will attract bacteria).

Use the teas of the watermelon seeds 2-3 times a day while on your watermelon-only cleanse.

How to use the rind

The rind is the outer shell of the watermelon.

You can eat the white/light green rind or juice it as well. The outer shell can also be juiced. Just make sure it's organic or well washed. Non-organic watermelon is usually heavily sprayed.

To increase the diuretic effect of watermelon, eat the white rind of the fruit (which is found just after the green, hard exterior rind or shell). Watermelon rind is used in Chinese medicine to help alleviate the symptoms of some cases of water retention, edema and jaundice due to its strong diuretic effect. [12][13]

How to pick the right watermelon

You can find watermelon at supermarkets worldwide. Local markets also carry them. Some retailers specialize in selling watermelon freshly squeezed. And you can find ground watermelon seeds and the rind at some herbal shops and some Asian markets.

Shopping for your watermelon

You can find watermelons in almost every market when in season. Most supermarkets carry them as well. The key is knowing how to spot the right watermelon.

Tips on how to identify a ripe and sweet watermelon

Look at the stem or where the stem was, and it should have sap dripping out (or it should be dried out). The tail of a watermelon has to be dried or shriveled — a strong green tail indicates that your watermelon was picked too soon and therefore the taste will not be as sweet or good. Look for dried tails for the best taste.

Look for a sunspot. A dark yellow or orange spot is preferred. The darker the spot, the better the flavor. A white spot means little or no taste.

Knock on it and listen. It should sound hollow, like there is space inside. It should not sound dense.

Other tips for picking a super sweet watermelon

If the watermelon has a uniform size and is heavy, it's sweet.

If it's elongated, it's watery.

A dark and dull watermelon is ripe.

A shiny skinned watermelon is unripe.

A watermelon with a large webbing on the skin is sweet and a watermelon with a small webbing on the skin is bland.

Pick the right gender of your melons.

Watermelons have genders. Male watermelons are more watery, taller and elongated, while female watermelons tend to be sweeter, round and stout.

Big is not better when picking a watermelon. The tastiest watermelons with the other points made above are average-sized. You don't want it too small or too big, but just average in size.

However, there's a small caveat to this tip. If the melon is heavier than it seems like it should be for its size, that's a good sign that it's a good one to pick.

Seeded or seedless watermelon

It's preferred that you use organic seeded watermelon but if you can't get seeded or organic, use seedless, for it still works and you can test it yourself. Now I'm not advocating genetically modified organisms (GMOs) but what I'm trying to tell you is that you use what you have available to you, and I advocate a no-excuses approach.

If you want to heal and you have seedless watermelon and you can't have the organic or seeded ones, then you use what you can get. There are many theories online about seedlessness, but they are just theories.

How to use the rind and peel of the watermelon for their health benefits

Cut off organic watermelon peels and dehydrate in a dehydrator or put them in the sun to dry out. When dry, you can grind and then store to be used as a herb in Chinese herbalism.

The ash of the dried rind of the watermelon can be applied on aphthous mouth ulcers for relief.[3]

*In some places, its rind is used to relieve diarrhea.[4]

TRADITIONAL APPLICATIONS

Watermelon has 92% of its volume as water and it's going to make you urinate. This is not a bad thing — consider it a flushing or cleansing and hydrating process. Watermelon is great for the urinary tract as well.

The excess urinating tends to reduce or stop once the body gets into balance (after a few days on watermelon only).

A glass of freshly squeezed watermelon juice has been used to relieve dizziness caused by sunstroke and vomiting.

Consume 2-4 cups of fresh watermelon two to three times a day to relieve excess thirst, bitter taste in the mouth, and the discharge of yellowish urine, bad breath, and pain in the urethra. It's also a remedy for hangovers.[5]

The juice of watermelon root has been used as a remedy to stop bleeding after an abortion.

Watermelon juice has been used as an antiseptic in the treatment of typhus fever.

Watermelon juice with cumin is a refreshing and hydrating drink. It is a good remedy to use in cases of painful gonorrhea, difficult urination, urinary tract infections, liver congestion and general inflammation.

It's also used in the treatment of diabetes in Chinese medicine: Take 30 grams of the skin of both a watermelon and winter melon and steam both in filtered water and then serve. This is to be done 3 times a day.

Eat 2-4 cups of watermelon 1-2 times a day to help reduce a fever that causes thirst and dry mouth; for an uneasy stomach that feels hot; and for a bitter taste in the mouth with bad breath.

To help relieve painful and yellow urine problems, eat 2-4 cups of fresh watermelon 2-3 times a day.

To remedy a hangover, eat 2-4 cups of fresh watermelon or take 60 grams of the skin and steam it in in water and serve.[9]

To treat hypertension, diabetes, and nephritis, boil 50 grams of dry watermelon peels in spring or distilled water and drink it as a tea.[10]

CAUTIONS:

Eat and don't juice if you have kidney filtration issues or swelling of any kind.

Watermelon is very hydrating and if you have swelling tendencies eat it and don't juice it to allow a slower digestion period.

Don't use watermelon if you have frequent urination.

Consume watermelon alone.

According to Chinese medicine, eating watermelon 30-60 minutes before a meal cleans the stomach and removes illnesses.[15, 11]

Its seeds are used traditionally to lessen the symptoms of mild bladder inflammation.

It is also used in Chinese herbal medicine for erectile dysfunction (ED) as well as skin conditions like acne.

It's used to remedy blood sugar issues like diabetes as well as water retention (edema).

Watermelon seed tea (Catullus vulgaris) is used in eclectic (early North American herbal medicine) medicine as a diuretic.

It can be used in cases of weak or slow urine (prostate inflammation).

Watermelon is great for kids. The seeds as an infusion (made as a tea) have traditionally been used for relieving the pain that occurs from the difficulty of the passage of urine as it stimulates the flow. When infants cry with every urination and their diaper is stained yellow, this remedy has been used to correct the condition.

It's also used for relieving bladder and urinary organs especially with conditions that are accompanied with the feeling of urine being constricted and/or backache from the passage of stones, urates and phosphates gravels.

It has been shown very useful for relief during the active stage of cystitis.[15] [16]

What if you have no watermelon where you live? Or if it's not watermelon season?

You might be reading this book and it might not be the season for watermelon but you still want to go on a cleanse. Well, you can still do it by substituting any other melon with watermelons.

Here are the basic types of melons you can sometimes find in a store or market:

Ananas
Apollo
Autumn Sweet Melon
Bailan Melon
Banana Melon
Bitter Melon
Canary Melon
Camouflage Melon
Cantaloupe (American)
Cantaloupe (European)
Casaba Melons
Casabanana
Charentais Melon
Crane Melon
Crenshaw Melon
Cucamelon
Galia Melons
Gac Melon
Golden Langkawi Melon

Golden Prize Melon
Hami Melon
Honey Globe Melon
Honeydew Melon
Horned Melon
Jade Dew Melon
Kantola Melon
Korean Melon
Maroon Cucumber
New Century Melon
Santa Claus Melon
Select Rocket Melon
Sky Rocket Melon
Sprite Melon
Sugar Melon
Ten Me Melon
Valencia Melon
Watermelon
Winter Melon

Fun fact: Did you know that the sweetest melon is cantaloupe?

EXTENDING THE 5 DAY CLEANSE

You need more than 5 days to cleanse the body. 5 days are a good period to lose some weight and give your digestive system a rest but some people might want to extend it for up to 3 cycles as follows:

Do 5 days of watermelon only cleanse.

Take 1-2 days off and use a mixed fruit diet. In this phase you can have any fruit you want. After 1-2 days go back to the watermelon only cleanse.

Do another 5 days of a watermelon only cleanse.

Take 1-2 days off and use a mixed fruit diet. In this phase you can have any fruit you want. After 1-2 days go back to the watermelon only cleanse.

Do a final 5 days of a watermelon only cleanse.

Transition out of the watermelon only cleanse with 1-2 days of mixed fruit diet and raw veggies. It has to be at least 80% fruits. Veggies are too bulky and slow the digestive process down. Use green drinks rather than eating raw veggies. In this phase you can have any fruit you want.

So you are doing three cycles of 5 days watermelon only cleanse, each phase is cycled with 1-2 days of mixed fruit eating.

Accelerate The Cleanse By Adding Some Dry Fasting

Don't add the dry fasting until you have done at least 14 days of watermelon only.

What is dry fasting?

Dry fasting is so beneficial to your body and organs, but only when done properly. If you are new to dry fasting please do not rush into it. Do thorough research and make sure your body is ready for what it is about to endure.

Dry fasting means no food and no water for an extended period of time be it 12 hours, 24 hours or even 72 hours or more. These longer periods of time should be off limits for beginners. Start slow and steady with an 8 hour long dry fast and gradually work your way up to 10 or 12. This is how to heal and strengthen your organs to be able to endure longer fasting periods, which means longer healing periods for your body.

You must always remember to break your dry fast with freshly squeezed watermelon juice, and nothing else. We use fruit juices because they are much less obstructive than fruits themselves and they are easier on your digestive organs. You may follow up with fresh watermelons after you've used watermelon juice to break your fast.

The best way to dry fast is to do it intermittently; meaning dry fast for 14 to 16 hours out of your day (once you've built your tolerance) then break it with fruit juices, eat some solid fruits and repeat this daily.

Always make sure you go on a 100% fruit diet for a week or two before you start your fast. This prepares your body to heal but cleaning up the digestive system, makes the lymph flow easier to the kidneys in preparation for acidic elimination.

The protocol for a dry fast with the watermelon would look like this:

Day 1. 12-14 hour dry fast, then follow with watermelon juice and then 30 minutes later actual watermelon to eat.
Day 2. Watermelon all day
Day 3. 12-14 hour dry fast, and then follow with watermelon juice and then 30 minutes later actual watermelon
Day 4. Watermelon all day
Day 5. 12-14 hour dry fast, then follow with watermelon juice and then 30 minutes later actual watermelon
Day 6: Watermelon all day
Day 7. 12-14 hour dry fast, and then follow with watermelon juice and then 30 minutes later actual

WHAT FRUITS TO EAT ON THE 1-2 DAYS OF MIXED FRUITS

There are certain categories of fruit and it is good to know what they are and how to use them together. These categories are: Sweet fruits, sub acid fruits, fatty fruits and acidic fruits.

The sweet fruit Category has some of the world's most popular fruits, like the Banana, Date, Fig, Sapote, Persimmon, Cherimoya, Carob, Mammea, Plantain, Sapodilla, Sugar Apple, etc. Not only are these fruits luscious, these fruits are high in nutrient density. These fruits carry enough energy in them to get you through your day-to-day life; busy lifestyles and intense exercise regimes included.

All of these fruits can be paired with all other fruits with the exception of acidic fruits and melons. They are also excellent with leafy greens and celery.

Acid fruits are exceptionally high in water content and tend to be low in calories, not to mention they taste amazing. Some of these fruits include Blackberry, Orange, Passion Fruit, Strawberry, Tangerine, Tomato (technically a fruit), Ugli Fruit, Grapefruit, Acerola Cherry, Grapefruit, Pineapple, just to mention a few. Low calorie fruits like oranges and grapefruits should be used by anyone in a hurry to lose weight, as opposed to calorie dense fruits, like the banana or avocado.

Even though these delicious fruits don't pair well with fruits from the Sweet category, they go well with everything else, including celery and leafy greens.

For the sub acid fruit category the following fruits are included: Peach, Pear, Apricot, Blackberry, Apple, Papaya, Raspberry, Ugli Fruit, Blueberry, Grape, Cherry, Mango, Mulberry, Nectarine, Tamarillo, Guava, and many many more. These fruits are also low in calories for the most part. Sub Acid fruits pair well with celery, lettuce, and all non-sweet fruits. Eat as many as you please!

It is no surprise that Melons have a category to themselves. Although the majority of people say that melons shouldn't be combined with other fruits because it will cause "melon belly", be your own judge because there are still some success stories about combining melons with other high-water fruits and veggies.

The Fat category includes Avocado's, Durians, Coconuts, Akee and so many more. Although fats are vital for the body to be able to manage its hormones and other critical functions, they will also start to disrupt our health when we consume them in large quantities. They will eventually start blocking the uptake of sugar from the bloodstream into the cells.
This is why consuming too many fatty fruits will bring about high blood sugar levels, which can lead to diabetes, candida, and several other ailments you do not want.

Here is the summary

1. Change the diet- By using the watermelon cleanse – it is 2-3 cups of fresh watermelon a meal and there are 3 to 5 meals a day
2. Use the herbs to clean and strengthen the structure and function of the cells
3. Open all elimination channels- get acids that cause health issues out of the body
4. Give it time- 5 days is a good cleansing period but you may or can extend it depending on your goals.

AFTER THE 5 DAY CLEANSE TRANSITION BACK

This is assuming you are using this cleanse for 5 days only. If you are using it longer simply cycle the 5 day cleanse as I illustrated above.

How to transition back: when you are done with the 5 days you should add soft fruits to the diet like berries, bananas or any fruit that is soft. You can also add green drinks. Do this for a day and then gradually add salads and then after 2 days some cooked alkaline vegan foods back to the diet.

It is advisable not to eat heavy cooked foods after a cleanse as the body is cleaner and more sensitive and you don't want to dump heavy obstructive and mucus forming foods into the body. (Protein and starches).

WHAT IS A HEALING CRISIS?

When it comes to healing with fruits, you have to be aware of the healing crisis that will come with your detox. You're going to feel and see the effects of toxins coming out of you. You may experience flu like symptoms, joint pain, irritability, muscle cramps, unusual fatigue or headaches.

Just remember that this is only temporary. This is the fruit detoxing your body of all waste and toxins in it. It's okay to visit a doctor if you feel worried, but healing crises are normal on a cleanse.

When you get through your healing crisis, everything tends to improve. This includes your health, your skin, and your hair. Lots of people experience energy that feels as though it has no bounds.

My advice to you is to have mental strength and knowledge about what you are doing and why you are doing it. So long as you keep in mind that you're detoxing for the sake of your health, you will get through your healing crisis.

If you find detox symptoms too much to bear, you can slow your detox down by eating a raw salad. If you want to stop your detox, eating cooked vegetables will do the trick.

Life after a cleanse

How to have a diet that will help you thrive. It makes no sense to continue eating the foods that cause obstructions of energy flow. These are animal products (including dairy) and starches (potatoes, flour, wheat, pasta and rice etc.).

I understand that we all have our "cheat" days where we eat foods we love that are bad for us. However these foods should be minimal and not a big part of our daily diet. If you eat the wrong foods (even a little) consistently every day its negative effects accumulate and will soon manifest as a health issue.

Foods you can have raw or cooked after your cleanse. It's called the mucusless diet or alkaline vegan diet.

A healthy diet should be 70% raw vegan / high fruit and the rest cooked alkaline vegan as shown below. You can use the list below to make your favorite foods.

In general the less cooked the food the better. Bake, sauté or steam your veggies are the best choices - try to avoid fried or grilled foods.

Recipes

There are so many alkaline vegan recipes on YouTube. Simply search for it using tis search keywords
"Vegan Alkaline Food Recipes"

Here is the list of what you can use in an alkaline diet.

Vegetables

Artichokes
Asparagus (tips)
Bamboo Shoots
Broccoli
Beetroots
Bell Peppers
Brussels Sprouts
Cabbages
Carrots
Cauliflowers
Celery
Chard
Chayote
Chicory
Chives
Collard Greens
Cucumbers

Dandelions
Dills
Dulce
Eggplant
Endives
Garlic
Green Beans
Green Olives
Green Peas
Greens (leafy)
Horseradish
Jerusalem Artichokes
Kak
Kelp
Leeks
Lettuces
Mustard Greens
Okra
Onions
Oyster plants
Parsley
Parsnips
Peas (fresh)
Peppers
Radishes
Rutabagas
Sea Veggies
Spinach
Summer squash
Sweet Potatoes
Swiss chard
Tomatoes
Turnips
Watercress
'Wheat grass
Wild Greens
Zucchini

Alkaline Fruits
All of them are alkaline and healing

Oils & Fats

Avocado Oil
Coconut Oil
Flax Oil
Hemp Seed Oil
Olive Oil
Safflower Oil
Sesame Oil

Sprouts

Alfalfa
Alfalfa Sprouts
Amaranth Sprouts
Barley Grass
Broccoli Sprouts
Dog Crass
Fenugreek
Sprouts
Kamut Crass
Kamut Sprouts
Lemon Crass
Millet Sprouts
Mung Bean
Sprouts
Oat Crass
Quinoa Sprouts
Shave Crass
Spelt Sprouts
Wheat Grass

Grains, Cereals & Breads

Amaranth
Buckwheat
Kamut
Millet
Quinoa
Spelt
Sprouted Breads
Sprouted Tortillas
Yeast-Free
Breads

Beans & Legumes are all moderately acidic and should be limited as treats or preferably avoided.

Nuts and Seeds

Almond Butter
Almonds
Caraway Seeds
Cumin Seeds
Fennel Seeds
Hemp Seeds
Pumpkin Seeds
Sesame Seeds
Sunflower Seeds
Drinks
Alkaline Water (not higher than 8 ph)
Barley Grass
Coconut water
Fresh Lemon
Lime Water
Fresh Veg Juices
Green Drinks
Green Tea
Herbal Tea
Wheatgrass Juice

Dairy & Meat- these are all acidic and should be avoided at all cost.

Condiments & Spices

(Unfermented Soy)
Almond Butter
Bee Pollen
Bragg Aminos
Chili Pepper
Cinnamon
Curry Powders
Ginger
Guacamole (freshly made)
Herbs (all)
Lemon Juice
Lime Juice

Sea Salt
Oriental
Vegetables
Daikon
Dandelion Root
Kombu
Maitake
Reishi
Sea Vegetables
Shitake
Umeboshi

Here is what I recommend as a long-term diet or long-term lifestyle change:

Breakfast: always fruit juices, preferably after 11 am.
Breakfast is not the most important meal; that's an advertising slogan and a lie. It's dangerous, as the body is cleaning or in a state of fast and should not be interrupted with a heavy meal.

Lunch: a big green salad, smoothies or green drinks.

Dinner: steamed veggies or cooked alkaline veggies; limit starches. You should focus on the list I gave you above. These foods are alkaline and mucus-free.

If you use the diet above as your baseline on a day-to-day basis, even if you do slip up, you will be far ahead in health and vitality.

Using herbs outside of a cleanse?

You can use herbs to help the structure and function of cells in your body outside of a cleanse. I always recommend that you address the fabulous five as I discussed above. I will list the herbs found in the fabulous 5 below.

PART 2: USING HERBS TO GET BETTER

I wrote this book to be an action book. I also wrote it to be effective on its own. Almost everyone who tries the 5 day cleanse is going to drop pounds. And is going to have a great cleanse and detoxification.
Why? It's cleansing to the organs, it gives the major systems a clean up and rest and opens up the channels of elimination.

However there are people whose glands and organs have been compromised from years of eating acidic foods and those people need the help of herbs. When you can't lose weight, it is often due to acidosis (the body will retain fat and water to buffer metabolic acids or waste it can't get rid of). The body will also use cholesterol and alkaline minerals and fats to bind to acids. This can make you retain weight that just won't go away.

The average human body and especially the colon is loaded with stagnant mucus, fecal matter, undigested and putrid foods- these wastes accumulation are a result of an acidic diet and a poisonous environment. This accumulated waste tends to stick to the wall of the colon (mucoid plaque) forcing the body to gain weight and it also tends to get released into our blood which then poisons our entire system.

The result is we tend to get sick, bloated and unhealthy.

If you don't digest your foods (pancreas and stomach), assimilate your foods (small intestines), utilize your foods (adrenals via metabolizing sugar; neurotransmitter production for peristalsis and steroid production and mineral utilization) and eliminate your food (excrete digestive waste), your body isn't going to be functioning properly

In such cases, we always use herbs to help clean and strengthen the function of cells. Herbs clean and help the structure and function of cells.

WHY DO WE USE HERBS IN REGENERATIVE DETOXIFICATION?

The use of herbs is a crucial part of healing the human body. Herbs work by cleansing and regenerating. Where medication deposits chemicals in the body, herbs come in and remove it.

And as herbs have not been hybridized by man, they hold all their nutritive and electrical properties.

From a spiritual point of view, herbs have consciousness; they know which body part or tissue to go to once consumed. They have consciousness that unites with the consciousness of the human cell, and this encourages the cell to function as it was originally designed to do.

Herbs are tissue specific, meaning that there are herbs for every part of the human body. When the plant is ingested, the compounds of the plant work synergistically to improve the functions of cells and the human body as a whole.

Herbs are used to address the root cause of health issues, while medications are used to treat symptoms. The problem is that you can't heal by treating symptoms; true healing and rebuilding comes from addressing the root cause of a health issue.

In short, herbs clean, strengthen, repair and rebuild cells, tissues, organs and glands and allow proper function of the human body.

The Fabulous 5 herbs

When it comes to detoxification, I like to use herbs that address the kidneys, the bowels, the adrenals, and the endocrine and lymphatic systems. I call these "fabulous 5" herbs, as they do a fabulous job of creating good health for the body.

Even if you feel your thyroid, adrenals, kidneys, bowels and endocrine glands don't need help, you should still make use of these herbs. They give you that extra optimization in healing and detoxification.

By using herbs, you are going to be able to experience the power of nature in its ability to optimize the health of the human body. You can also combine herbs for a synergistic effect on the body and its cells. There are herbs for every part of the human body, and we the human species have not even discovered all of them yet.

Here are the fabulous 5 (Herbs for the adrenals, kidneys, lymph system, endocrine and bowels) and the herbs that come under it.

For the adrenal glands:

Chaste Tree Berry
Cleavers Herb
Dandelion Root & Leaf
Eleuthero Root
Ho Shou Wu Root
Holy Basil
Juniper Berry
Kelp
Parsley (whole)
Rhodiola Root
Saw Palmetto Berry
Wild Yam Root

For the lymphatic system:

Cleavers Herb
Echinacea Root
Plantain Leaf
Poke Root
Prickly Ash Bark
Red Root
White Oak Bark

For the kidneys:

Cordyceps
Corn Silk

Buchu
Uva Ursi
Cleavers herb
Nettle seed or leaf
Couch Grass Root
Dandelion Leaf
Goldenrod
Horsetail Herb
Juniper Berry
Parsley Leaf
Stinging Nettle Leaf

Herbs for the endocrine glands:

The endocrine glands here include the thyroid, parathyroid, hypothalamus, pituitary, adrenals, pineal, ovaries and testes.

Astragalus Root
Bee Propolis Powder
Chaste Tree Berry
Eleuthero Root
Ho Shou Wu Root
Kelp Fronds Powder
Parsley (whole)
Prickly Ash Bark
Saw Palmetto Berry
Suma Root
Wild Yam Root

For the stomach and bowels

Cape Aloe Leaf
Cascara Sagrada Bark
Fennel Seed
Gentian Root
Ginger Root
Plantain Leaf

Slippery Elm Bark
White Oak Bark
Wild Yam Root

It is best to have a combination of herbs for each gland or organ. For instance, you can have corn silk, couch grass, dandelion leaf and goldenrod combined to make a tea or tincture versus just using dandelion root for the kidneys. This is because herbs work synergistically. You need to be an herbalist to understand how to combine these herbs, but I am showing you the best herbs I know for each major system, gland or organ. As an herbalist, I already have the combinations done for you on my website. Use the resources link below to get them already made for you.

HOW TO COMBINE THE HERBS WITH THE WATERMELON ONLY CLEANSE

The best way to use the herbs is in tincture or tea form. Tinctures are more potent, but ideally use both, as the teas allow you to take in more water with an electrical and nutritive touch to it. You want to make use of the herbs I just listed for you. Make them into teas and drink them all day. Use the tincture form to get more plant essence delivered to your cells. Teas, for instance, will give you approximately 10-15% of plant essences, but a tincture extracts about approximately 90% of the plant essence, so it's more potent and effective.

Here is how I would use them:

Use the tinctures of the herbs 2-3 times a day, 30 minutes before or after a watermelon only meal.

Use the dried herbs as a tea 2-3 times a day. Make a big pot of herb tea and drink it all day- the act of dipping it all day is called micro dosing and it's very effective.

Stay consistent with the herbs and you will get benefits from them.

Q: Can I use only a few of these herbs?

A: Yes, you can, but it's preferable to get them in combination as a tincture and use them all, as that offers a synergistic effect to the cells of the body. You can find good formulas on my website (see the resource section at the end of the book)

Open all the elimination channels to maximize the cleanse.

When it comes to good health, we need to eat the right foods to supply the cells with the energy they need, but we also need to remove the waste from cell activity. To help the body get rid of metabolic waste, we can take steps to open the 4 elimination channels of the body.

Lack of elimination leads to accumulation of metabolic waste, toxins and mucus buildup. All this in turn affects health.

The main elimination channels are the kidneys, the skin, the lungs and the bowels.

Skin – Help the skin eliminate waste by sweating a lot. Use a steam sauna and/or walk 30 minutes a day at the least. Be sure to stay hydrated as you do this on a daily basis – especially these 7 days. A 30-minute walk will do wonders for your weight loss efforts as well. Use a skin brush or dry brush to brush your skin on a daily basis. You can also take steam baths. Find any way to sweat without overexerting yourself. Do not perform any high intensity workouts, as these activities generate lots of lactic acid and acidic waste, and we want to minimize acid buildup in and accelerate acid removal from the body.

Here are the best herbs to use for the skin:
Chickweed Herb,
Poke Root,
Red Clover,
Burdock Root,
Oregon Grape,
Chamomile Flower,
It's best to use all these in a tincture as opposed to loose herbs as a tea.

You can also use the following herbs to promote sweating:
Yarrow Flower, Boneset, Red Raspberry Leaf, Elder Flower, Peppermint leaf, Hyssop herb

Clear the lungs – Use deep breathing exercises and use herbs for the lungs in the form of a tea or tincture, as they help to loosen and relieve congestion in the chest. **Good herbs for the lungs are:**

Mullein
Slippery Elm Bark
Pleurisy Root
Elecampane
Horsetail
Fenugreek
Wild Cherry
Coltsfoot
Lobelia

CLEAN YOUR BOWELS

Use herbs for the bowels (the herbs I listed above) as well as enemas; the undiluted lemon only diet will help you eliminate stagnant waste from your bowels. Experts claim there are pounds of fecal matter on our bowel walls. There is also mucoid plaque (a rubbery mucus) that coats our small intestines and prevents proper absorption. This mucoid plaque is from eating protein and starches, which tend to stick like glue to the bowel walls and create ill health.

Using herbs for the bowels will help remove this waste and clean and strengthen the structure and function of cells in the bowel walls.

Make use of enemas in this cleanse on a daily basis to help remove clogged fecal matter. Lemon juice, wheat grass or just plain distilled water is all you need for the enema fluid. You will need an enema bag, which you can get online. Do not use the chemicals that often come in enema bags; rinse the bag with distilled water before you use it.

Use herbs to address digestion, which means you will want to make use of herbs for the liver, gallbladder and pancreas. Here are a few good suggestions:

Panax ginseng
Gymnema sylvestre
Cedar berry
Fenugreek
Bitter melon
Turmeric - Curcuma
Milk thistle seeds
Ganoderma
picrorhiza kurroa

Of these, milk thistle is a liver trophorestorative and strengthens the liver. A trophorestorative for the pancreas is Gymnema leaves.
A trophorestorative for the gallbladder is globe artichoke (don't use if your bile duct is obstructed).

To clean the kidneys, you will want to make use of the herbs I mentioned above. You can also use a castor oil pack and place it onto of the kidneys (lower back region) to reduce inflammation and soothe them.

Gentle and soft massages to the kidneys (lower back) will also help tremendously.

I just shared the very best herbs and plants that I know of to get the cells clean and strong in combination with the diet.

While on the watermelon cleanse, you can make use of herbs to help your kidneys in certain ways. These herbs are not for treating, but are for cleaning and strengthening cells. So if you need treatment, see your doctor.

Here are herbs to target specific issues of the kidneys:

To strengthen the kidneys, you will want to make use of nettle seed. It's a kidney trophorestorative.

And nettle leaf is a great kidney antioxidant and detoxifier.

Nettle root is great for the kidneys and has other therapeutic properties, but is also an inhibitor of the aromatase enzyme in prostate tissue. It has been reported that clinical symptoms of prostatic hyperplasia were improved with nettle root.

The best herb to use for kidney infections is agropyron.

Use uva ursi for cystitis.

Use chimaphila and piper methysticum for painful urination.

Use zea (corn silk) for alkaline urine.

Herbs for kidney stones include Phyllanthus niruri. Common name: Chanca piedra - the stone breaker.[17]

Bonus

If you have low energy, you will want to try this.

There are four reasons why you might experience low energy levels.

The first reason would be a neurological issue. Neurological weaknesses will affect your energy levels and cause fatigue.

The second reason is your adrenals. The adrenals are responsible for sugar metabolism, so when your sugar levels fluctuate a lot, it will cause your energy levels to do the same.

The third reason for fatigue could be a weak thyroid. Thyroid issues, more specifically hypothyroidism, will throw off your metabolic rate; this will affect your energy levels too.

The fourth reason could be fungus. Fungus overgrowth or candida can eventually spread all the way to the head region and affect your energy levels as well.

To address these, you will want to use the watermelon-only cleanse and add herbs to target the adrenals, thyroid, the nervous system and fungus.
Below are formulas you can use as a tea or tincture. I prefer tinctures and I prefer that you use all the herbs in the formulas. If you can't get all of them, use what you can get from the formula.

Adrenals:

My favorite herb for the adrenals would be licorice root as it's an adrenal trophorestorative. What are the benefits of trophorestoratives?
The "trophic" condition represents a system's or tissue's vital capacity in the body.
So licorice is a good herb to boost the vitality of your adrenals. Don't use licorice root if you have high blood pressure.
Herbs to use for adrenals:
Bupleurum
Panax
Ginseng
Wild Yam

Adrenal formula 2

American Ginseng, Ashwagandha, Astragalas, Cordyceps, Gynostemma, Holy Basil, Licorice, Rhodiola, Schisandra, Siberian Ginseng.

Thyroid herbs and formula

Kelp is a thyroid trophorestorative.
Other good herbs to use for the thyroid are:
Ashwagandha, Bacopa, Barberry, Bladderwrack, Guggulu, , Oregon Grape, Pashanbheda, Rhodiola, Triphala.

To fight fungal overgrowth, uses these herbs:

Barberry, Echinacea, Garlic, Golden Thread Root, Goldenseal Root, Myrrh, Pau D'Arco, Reishi Mushroom, Sweet Annie.

Bonus 2

How to use herbs to fight knee pain

These herbs are well known to relieve knee pain:

Althea - Marshmallow plant.
Chamomile (Matricaria chamomilla L.).
Chelidonium majus, commonly known as greater celandine (good for relief of right knee pain). Cinchona succirubra (relaxes the ligaments and relieves pain).
Helianthemum Canadense - Frostweed - this is for relieving swelling of the knee.
Nymphaea - water lily (strengthen week knees).
Polygonatum - Solomon seal - lubricates the joints.
Sambucus nigra – elderberry - relieves joint pain.
Symphytum - comfrey is great at relieving pain and stiffness and in improving physical functioning of joints.

Here is a formula to use:

40% of Polygonatum
10% each of:
Chamomile (Matricaria chamomilla L.)
Symphytum
celandine (good for relief of right knee pain) Cinchona succirubra
Nymphaea - water lily
Sambucus nigra
Symphytum - comfrey

You can use these as a tincture, loose herbs or teas.

FREQUENTLY ASKED QUESTIONS (FAQs)

Q: I am swelling up on watermelon. What can I do?

A: Stop the cleanse. Here is why it may happen.
The watermelon-only cleanse is very astringent as its pulls at lymph and it helps in moving the lymph system, so if your kidneys are not filtering out waste, parts of the body can swell up a bit. A solution is to make use of dry fasting and try different fruits like grapes and other berries. I would not be forcing the body and staying on the watermelon cleanse, because when you have swelling, it means your lymph system is congested and it means your kidneys are also not filtering properly.

Q: So what happens after the five-day detox?

A: When you are done with the detox, I recommend that you go to a balanced diet. I prefer an alkaline vegan diet. This is a diet that is high in raw veggies mixed with cooked alkaline food. You can have some cooked now and then and that's how you maintain the results of the cleanse. I recommend you don't go on a cooked diet of protein and starches, as this leads to obstructions and health issues arising.

Q: Why 5 days?

A: Five days is a nice cleanse. It's enough to give you a taste of the effectiveness of the fruits to cleanse the body.

Q: Can I heal just one part of my body? For example, my liver?

A: No. The body is a whole entity and functions as a whole and everything affecting its parts affects the whole organism. You need to heal the whole body to fully heal your liver (not treat but heal).

Q: How much and how often should I eat?

A: It's best to have small frequent meals every two hours. When I say small, I mean one or two cups. Don't overeat and don't under eat. You want the belly to be half full always because you're eating nutrient-dense rich foods. You don't need a lot of food but at the same time don't starve yourself. Eat until satisfied; never overeat.

Q: What if I can't get the herbs?

A: If you can't get herbs, go ahead with the cleanse and use watermelon only. Use no excuses. The goal is to get you better.

Q: I am too thin. Should I do a cleanse (detox)?

A: Detoxification is like driving your own car. You must know when to step on the gas (accelerate the detox with fruits and dry fasting), slow down (raw greens) or step on the brakes (cooked veggies). You must listen to your body. Being thin does not mean you don't have obstructions of lymph and mucus, and in fact often you have malabsorption issues that make you thinner than you should be. Your job is to remove obstructions at your own pace.

Q: Why do we use herb?

A: Herbs are used to help the structure and function of cells in the body. They contain phytonutrients that help cells and the body function better.

Herbs are designed for the human body to help clean and strengthen the structure and function of cells of the body. So it's about optimizing the structure and function of cells.

Herbs are tissue-specific. There are herbs for every single part of the body. If you want to strengthen the liver, there are herbs for that.

Q: Why use the fabulous 5 herbs?

A: These herbs cover the adrenal glands, lymphatic system, endocrine glands, bowels and kidneys. These parts of the body are essential to cover during a cleanse.

When detoxing the body, I like to use the fabulous five always as the base and then I add to this based on what I need extra help with.

For instance, if you have a liver issue, you want to use the fabulous 5 herbs and liver and pancreas herbs.

If you have kidney issues, you want to use the fabulous 5 herbs and extra kidney herbs like nettle seed tea.

Let's say you want to fix the brain. Then you use the fabulous 5 plus the neurological one tincture because it strengthens the brain and the nervous system.

If you want a stronger spleen, then use the fabulous 5 and lymphatic and spleen herbs.

That's a basic and general overview of how to use herbs to help the body get better. Herbalism is a practice that requires years of study, but you can still derive benefits from herbs if you have a basic understanding of how to use them.

Q: Why can't I have cooked foods on a cleanse?

A: Cooked foods are not healing foods. You have to understand that when you cook food, you destroy and alter chemistry and this is harmful to the human body. Having cooked food now and then is okay for a balanced lifestyle but it's not going to improve your health if you are sick.
You need to eat foods that give you more energy than they take away through digestion.

Life begets life and death begets death.

If you are eating dead foods, you are robbing yourself of vitality slowly. It leads to an obstructive state in the body, which leads to ill health. Raw fruits and veggies are superior as they are as nature designed them, complete and balanced with the right ratios of nutrients, enzymes and healing properties.

Q: What's the best way to juice a watermelon?

A: Any juicer will do. I personally use a masticating juicer - mine is the Omega 8006, which is old, but I have used it without problems for 8 years.

Q: What if watermelon gives me nausea?

A: Use any other melon and if you still have an issue, use a mixed fruit diet with the fabulous 5 herbs.

Q: Is it okay to eat and not juice the melon?

A: Yes. You can do one or the other or both as well.

Q: Is there a limit to how much or how little to eat?

A: 2-4 cups per meal is sufficient for most. However, eat small, frequent meals, and eat if hungry.

Q: If I eat the seeds, will I slow the detox?

A: No. The seeds are very beneficial, so chew them or use them in a tea. If you don't have the seeds, use the tincture (you can find it in the resource section).

Q: What can I combine with watermelon?

A: You should not combine foods on this cleanse. However, you can add limejuice or fresh mint for a change in taste.

Q: Eating a one-fruit (mono) diet is boring, isn't it?

A: It can be, but it's only for 5 days. It's a cleanse, and really a mono fruit diet makes your life simple. You don't need to think about what's for dinner - you save so much time - you don't have to worry about whether certain foods are allowed on this cleanse, as every meal is a mono fruit.

Q: Is organic watermelon a must or can I use a regular one?

A: Use organic seeded, but if you can't find organic seeded, use seedless organic. If no seedless organic, use conventional as it still does work as a cleanser.

Q: Can I just juice the watermelon? Is the juice a meal?

A: Juicing is a very strong detoxification tool, so be sure to go by how you feel. Small, frequent meals are best, and this includes juicing. Juicing is a meal, so have enough of it (just don't overdo it).

Q: I can't find seeded watermelons.

A: There is a misconception about hybrids. There is a big difference between a hybrid and GMO fruit. A hybrid is not necessarily GMO, especially if organic. All offer nutrition and healing. I just would not use GMO. In the world we live in, you can't always get seeded or non-hybrid (unless you live in the tropics or Asian countries), so you use what you can get. It's better than a diet of protein and starches. No excuses.

The paranoia of hybrids comes from Dr. Sebi's followers, but don't forget that Dr. Sebi healed himself personally on a water fast and herbs. The highest form of detox is a dry fast, then water fast, then fruit juices, then fruits, then green drinks, then raw veggies. Remember that healing is a "fasting experience."

Always safely test ideologies on yourself and see the truth for yourself. It's fruits, fasting and herbs for simplicity and healing power.

Q: Watermelons are not in season where I live. What can I use?

A: Use cantaloupe or honeydew for your 5-day cleanse. There is a list of all the melons you can use in the resource section.

Q: Can I drink water on this cleanse?

A: Yes you can. Use distilled or spring water. Don't use water from plastic bottles as they contain micro plastics in them.

Q: I have low energy. What can I use?

A: Licorice root tea and Chinese ginseng root (don't drink this before bed.)

Q: What if I cave in to temptation?

A: Restart the cleanse on the very next meal. Don't cancel the day.

Q: I can't make the changes. I have no self-discipline. What can I do?

A: Use this approach:

Breakfast after 11 am: fruits

Lunch: fruits

Dinner: cooked alkaline vegan

This will build success and you can eventually go on a 100% fruit diet.

Rest and get enough sleep.

Take walks, play a board game, go to bed early and meditate.

Q: How long can I store the juice?

A: One day, as after that, it loses most of its nutrients and enzymes.

Q: Can I buy store-made juice?

A: No, unless it's unpasteurized and made and consumed the same day.

Q: I am bored with watermelon. What can I do?

A: Add these to the list:

Mint and lime

Q: I am going through an emotional detox. What can I do?

A: Meditate and let your emotions out.

Q: I get red stools when I eat watermelon. Why?

A: This can happen because the pulp of the watermelon will often pass through the small and large intestines without being fully digested and can appear as red stools. You can always strengthen the pancreas and gut overall with liver, pancreas and bowel herbs.

Q: I am on the watermelon cleanse and herbs. I am getting detox symptoms. Am I detoxing too fast?

A: You got detox symptoms such as headaches, cold and flu, slight worsening of symptoms. These are detox symptoms. They're not from the herbs but the whole process of cleansing or detoxing. It's toxins and stagnant mucus being dislodged. You can slow down the detox and add steamed veggies. You can also take steps to clean your sinuses (often a cause of headaches) such as: use a Neti pot with eucalyptus oil, ear candling, etc.

You can also use reduce the dosage of herbs used to slow the detox process.

Q: Is it okay to use nettle leaf tea for my kidneys as opposed to nettle seed and can I dry the seeds from my watermelon and use them to make tea?

Yes, you can use any part of the nettle plant. Nettle leaf is a kidney detoxifier; nettle seed is a kidney builder.

Q: I'm a deliveryman and driver with lots of physical activity and need energy to keep up with my routine. Will I have all the energy I need thru this cleanse by eating only watermelons?

A: Yes, you will get all the energy you need from this cleanse. You are consuming one of the most electrifying and energetic foods on the planet. To get the most energy, consume small frequent meals (every two hours).

Next, use an adrenal restorative herbal combination with the following herbs: Panax ginseng, Licorice root, Wild yam and Bupleurum.

Q: While on the 5-day cleanse, do I need to rest? Can I do this with my busy lifestyle looking after two toddlers?

A: You don't need extra rest, although resting always helps in detoxification. So rest when you can with short naps and a good night's sleep.

Q: How do I get rid of cravings during the cleanse?

A: Cravings are due to weak adrenals and parasites. There is also a mental hindrance. I would use antimicrobial and parasite herbs to fight parasites and use herbs for the adrenals to strengthen your adrenals (adrenals help with sugar metabolism; if you can't metabolize sugar properly, it ferments and attracts fungus). Also have small (1 cup) frequent meals every two hours to deal with the cravings.

Q: What can I do for the headaches during the cleanse?

A: Place a drop of organic essential peppermint oil on your temple (forehead) and also sniff the oil for 2-3 seconds for relief.

Q: For the watermelon seeds, once crushed and brewed with hot water for a tea, do we need to filter it and drink the water or not filter it? Can I eat those crushed seeds in the tea?

A: It's up to you, but the seeds are edible. Chew it well before you swallow to help with digestion.

Q: What are the benefits of dandelion?

A: The root is used for the liver and kidneys. The leaf is a good diuretic and is good for the kidneys.

Q: I'm wondering if squeezing lime on the watermelon is okay for the detox?

A: You can squeeze lime or lemons on the watermelon and even throw in some fresh mint as well!

Q: Can I juice and eat the watermelon during the cleanse?

A: Yes, you can use both. Just make sure it's freshly squeezed and consumed within a few hours (maximum 24 hours).

Q: Since I started the detox, I have noticed that my legs, ankles and feet are swollen. Why is this happening?

A: Watermelon has a very high water content 92%. Swelling indicates weak kidney filtration and acidosis in the body.

To improve kidneys, use 14-to-16-hour dry fasts and eat (don't juice) your melons. If it persists, try another fruit like grapes or raw veggies until you strengthen your kidneys. Use herbs like nettle seed and leaves to help strengthen and cleanse your kidneys.

Q: I heard that watermelon is good for breasts. Why?

A: It has high levels of lycopene, which is an antioxidant with many health benefits such as sun protection, improved heart health and a lower risk of certain types of abnormal cell activity. With lycopene, you want to not supplement with it but get it from food sources like watermelon and other red or pink fruits. The lycopene in watermelon is amazing for the breast. It actually has the highest level of lycopene.

Q: Can I juice my watermelon ahead of time?

A: Fresh is always best. Ideally you shouldn't juice it until you are ready to drink it but if you have no other choice and just don't have the time, juice them for the day. 24 hours is the maximum you should store it as it loses its enzymes and nutrients the longer you store it.

Q: Can I use high pH or alkalizing water?

A: High pH or alkaline water I would not touch. Use it only to wash produce. Too high a pH is bad and high pH is not necessarily alkalizing. To alkalize you need nutrients. High pH water has no nutrients.

Q: I need a dessert on the cleanse. What can I have?

A: Watermelon ice lollies. Freeze your watermelon juice as an ice lolly.

Q: How do I stay accountable to myself?

A: Commit and stay away from family and friends that tempt you, rest, and get extra sleep.

Q: What if I am hypoglycemic?

A: Don't use this cleanse.

Q: How long does it take for the watermelon seeds to dry?

A: A day if sun dried or a few hours if you use a dehydrator.

Q: Are fruits and herbs a way to heal everything?

A: No, but they are a way to detox the body to a point where the body can self-heal. The body is the healer. Fruits and herbs are mere tools. As in natural healing, we don't label symptoms as diseases but rather obstructions to the flow of energy (blood flow, lymph flow and nerve flow).

Q: Getting healthy is expensive, as herbs and fruits are expensive.

A: You can start small with the following: Chaste Tree Berry, Dandelion Root, Holy Basil, Juniper Berry, Plantain Leaf, White Oak Bark, Prickly Ash Bark, Goldenrod, Corn Silk, Horsetail Herb. FYI, getting ill is way more expensive and health is priceless, so invest in your fruits and herbs and stop buying stuff you may not need.

Q: I woke up this morning and my shirt was drenched in sweat. I'm feeling weak, and my scalp itches. Why?

A: These are healing crises. Itching indicates fungus and toxins trying to come out. Use lymphatic and kidney herbs.

Q: My main reason for the detox is weight loss, yet I am having lots of cravings. What must I do?

A: Eat small, frequent meals and use antimicrobial herbs. I have these as parasites with tincture and antimicrobial tincture on my website. See the resources area. Also, work on the adrenals glands, as they handle sugar metabolism. Use adrenal herbs such as my adrenals restorative tincture.

Q: I keep getting cramps. How can I fix it?

A: Cramps will come but it's from weak adrenals and a calcium and magnesium imbalance. Have a banana and see. Use adrenal restorative tincture on my website. Herbs to use: Panax ginseng, Licorice root, Wild yam, and Bupleurum

Q: Why go on a cleanse?

A: We are eating the wrong foods: proteins, starches, cooked foods, processed foods and chemicals create obstructions in the human body. These obstructions are excess mucus and acids that block the flow of energy in the body. And fruits are the least obstructive foods you can eat, so when we are going on a cleanse to try and dislodge obstructions, we use the least obstructive foods, which are the fruits. Watermelon is one of the least obstructive and takes 20 minutes to digest.

The human body is not designed to eat complex chemical starches and proteins. These foods obstruct energy flow. The GI tract (gastrointestinal tract) is not meant to take in massive amounts of foods at a frequent rate.

Energy flow is defined as blood flow, lymph flow and nerve flow. If any of these are blocked, you're going to have a health issue.

So when you have a health issue, your goal is to unlock these energy flows.

Q: What are the energy flows?

A: They are blood flow, lymph flow and nerve flow. You need blood flow to feed the cells, nerve flow to communicate between the cells and lymph flow to remove waste from the cells. All those three have to be in good working order for good health.

The fruits are the only way you're going to be able to remove these obstructions, because fruits are astringent (they have drawing and pulling ability), and more importantly, they move the lymph system.

Fruits are also easy to digest, and the less the digestion process, the more energy is left over for healing and cleaning.

It is crucial that your gut remains empty and free of obstructions. Therefore you cannot be eating foods and piling on even more foods that are not being broken down into your GI tract.

Remember that a backed-up Gi tract leads to congestion, which leads to health issues.

Resources

We do carry all the herbs I mentioned above in tincture or tea form, the herbs are combined for you. You can see the herbs we have right here:
https://miraherbals.info/collections/product-for-health